Expectir
For New Moms

Introduction

I want to thank you and congratulate you for downloading the book, *"Expecting A Baby For New Moms"*.

When that home pregnancy test kit or blood test returns positive, your world spines off. Immediately, you start thinking of all the things you out to buy, all the ways you ought to prepare, and all the changes you will undergo.

Amidst the excitement, it is normal to feel panicky because the thought of carrying a baby to term, taking care of your health as well as the health of the baby and caring for a baby after birth is overwhelming.

The best way to prepare yourself for motherhood as well as pregnancy is to become knowledgeable. In this guide, **Expecting a Baby for New Moms**, we shall look at, and understand the trimesters and the changes you can expect to see as your pregnancy progresses. You will also learn about how to take care of your health and your baby's as well as how to prepare for labor and child birth.

Thanks again for downloading this book, I hope you enjoy it!

information is without contract or any type of guarantee assurance.

The trademarks that are used are without any consent, and the publication of the trademark is without permission or backing by the trademark owner. All trademarks and brands within this book are for clarifying purposes only and are the owned by the owners themselves, not affiliated with this document.

Table of Contents

What To Expect In The First Trimester

You can never be 100% certain that you are pregnant until you take a home pregnancy test or a blood test at your OB's office. To get the correct results, do the test after missing your menstrual period. A missed period does not necessarily mean you are pregnant, but it is one of the major signs indicating that you could be pregnant.

To count the duration of a pregnancy, we start from the first day of your last menstrual period up to the 37th-40th week. These 37-40 weeks further divide into three trimesters that last 13 weeks each.

The first trimester starts on the first week, which begins on the first day of your last menstrual period all through to the 13th week. During the first trimester, although your pregnancy may not show, your body is going through many internal changes as it seeks to accommodate the growing fetus.

To make this guide an easier read and comprehension, we shall divide each trimester into individual weeks. Here is what to expect in every week of the first trimester.

Week 1 And 2 Of Pregnancy

This is the week immediately after your last menstrual period. Here are the changes you should expect to see:

Changes In Your Body

At this time, there are no noticeable or physical changes in your body because you are actually not pregnant since no fertilization has occurred. Your uterus has shed its last month's unfertilized egg which is the process that just happened (menstruation). A new cycle which is the starting point of your pregnancy begins. Your period has just ended and you are getting ready for ovulation. For many women, this happens 11 to 19 days from the first day of their last menstrual period.

The first thing to happen is production of Follicle Stimulating Hormone (FSH) that stimulates the follicles to mature. Each follicle has an egg and only one follicle becomes dominant each month.

During the maturation process, the follicles produce two hormones called Progesterone and Estrogen; these hormones help repair and thicken the walls of the uterus. Estrogen triggers the production of Luteinizing hormone (LH). LH makes the most mature follicle, which has already become the egg, bursts through the ovarian wall about 24 to 26 hours after the LH surge. This process is the ovulation process.

Week 3

In your due date calendar, this is the third week of your pregnancy, but in real sense it is the first week because fertilization takes place during this week, which is also when you conceive. This explains why your due date will have 40weeks of pregnancy but you will only carry your baby for 38 weeks.

Changes In Your Body

Although your body still has no noticeable changes, you are pregnant. The uterus will produce more endometrium to provide a healthy environment for your baby to implant. During week three, some signs you should look out for include:

Fatigue: Because of the increased progesterone production, you may experience overwhelming tiredness. To prevent or reduce this feeling, use prenatal vitamins, eat a balanced diet, drink plenty of fluids, and rest when you can to keep your blood pressure high enough and supportive of the many activities going on in your body.

Implantation bleeding: During implantation, light vaginal bleeding may occur. This bleeding is normal and harmless; however, if you suspect and think you are pregnant, visit your doctor or OB because the bleeding may be something else such as an infection, ectopic pregnancy, or miscarriage.

Your Baby's Development

The egg stays in the fallopian tube for about 24 hours waiting for a sperm to fertilize it. One of the many sperms will fertilize an ovum and create a set of 46 chromosomes called a zygote.

After fertilization, the fertilized egg stays in the fallopian tube for 3 to 4 days and then travels from the fallopian tube towards the womb, dividing into more and more cells called morula. The morula will become the blastocyst that will end up in the womb and attach itself to the lining of the uterus where it will set up its residence for the next nine months. This is the process called implantation. The blastocyst divides into two parts:

1. The external part called the trophoblast that becomes the placenta.

2. The internal part called the inner cell mass that becomes the embryo.

At week three, it is possible to determine the sex of your baby depending on the chromosomes that fertilized the ovum. Out of the 46 chromosomes, only X chromosomes and Y chromosomes are important. All ova in a woman's body have X chromosome and all sperms have either X chromosome or Y chromosome.

If a Y chromosome fertilized the egg, you will be having a boy, and if an X chromosome fertilized the egg, your baby will be a girl. In addition, the genetic materials of the chromosomes will determine the skin color, hair color, eye color, height, and other features of your baby.

At this stage, your baby is an embryo and has 150 cells that will start to divide into three germ layers (gastrula) through a process called gastrulation. These layers are:

1. Endoblast or Endoderm

This is the innermost layer of an embryo; it forms when the cells migrate inward along the archenteron. Endoderm consists of flattened cells that become columnar and develop into the lining of the digestive system (except the pharynx, the terminal part of the rectum and the mouth that forms by involutions of the ectoderm), the respiratory system (except the nose), glands such as the pancreas, thymus, bladder, urethra, and thyroid.

2. Mesoderm

The mesoderm is the middle layer of an embryo between the endoderm and ectoderm. Mesoderm leads to the development of coelom where organs formed inside it can freely develop, move, and grow independently of the body. This layer develops into circulatory system, muscles, bones, cartilage, kidney, gonads, excretory system, inner skin layer, and outer covering. Tissues that come from the mesoderm layer are smooth muscles in the gut, red blood cells, skeletal muscle cells, cardiac muscle, and the tubule cells of the kidney.

3. Ectoderm

This is the outer most layer of an embryo; it forms from the embryo's epiblast. It develops into neural crest, neural tube, and surface ectoderm.

The neural crest develops into facial cartilage, teeth dentin, adrenal medulla, and the peripheral nervous system. The neural tube develops into the spinal cord, brain, retina, posterior pituitary, and motor neurons. The surface ectoderm develops into nails, hair, epidermis, eye lens, sebaceous glands, nose, and mouth epithelium.

Week 4

This is the second week since conception; you have missed your periods, right? If you want to be sure of your pregnancy, this is the right time to do it. Visit your obstetrician (OB) or buy an over the counter home test kit and follow the directions detailing how to use it.

Changes In Your Body

Your body will start producing Human Chorionic Gonadotropin (HGC) hormone, which can cause nausea. This can start as early as one week after conception. The higher the level of HCG in your body, the more sickly you will feel.

If you experience nausea symptoms, you can use ginger or lemon, something most new mothers-to-be find soothing. If this does not work for you, consult your doctor about vitamin B6 supplements that can alleviate nausea.

Your Baby's Development

In the fourth week of pregnancy, different organs are developing every day, the heart has started beating, and blood is beginning to pump. Your baby is 4 to 5 millimeters long, but your doctor might not be able to see it clearly.

Your baby (embryo) has developed two layers called the **hypoblast** and the **epiblast**.

Hypoblast is tissue formed from the inner cell mass that lies beneath the epiblast and consists of small cuboidal cells. Its key role is to aid the orientation of the embryonic axis and yolk sac formation. The yolk sac provides blood and guarantees effective exchange of gases, nutrients, and wastes until the placenta develops and takes over.

Epiblast forms from the inner cell mass, opposite the trophoblast, above the hypoblast and has columnar cells. It migrates far from the trophoblast, leaving a space in between them called the amniotic cavity that fills with amniotic fluid to protect the baby from shock.

Week four of pregnancy is when the chorion develops. Chorion is the outer membrane around the embryo that forms the fetal part of the placenta.

Week 5

You are one month and one week pregnant; an ultrasound will show that there is a baby in your womb.

Changes In Your Body

Your belly is yet to protrude and people around you will not tell if you are pregnant. The signs and symptoms you experienced in the previous week will still manifest and may be more persistent. At week five, some of the signs and symptoms you should expect include:

Backache, bloating, and cramps: These symptoms emanate from the growth of your uterus, and hormonal changes going on in your body. Most people mistake these symptoms with those common during the menstrual period and often, many women think that they are about to menstruate instead of thinking that they are pregnant.

These symptoms are normal and there is little you can do about the; however, if the backache and cramps are severe, seek medical attention.

Breast Changes: Your breasts will become swollen and tender because of the high production of estrogen and progesterone. Although these changes are similar to those you may experience a few days before your period, the difference is that the skin around your nipple becomes darker. Other than buying supportive right-sized bras, you cannot do much about these symptoms.

Constipation: The increased production of Progesterone will cause your digestion to slow down and you will start to experience indigestion or constipation because your stomach will not digest food as quickly as it normally does. Your digestion will assume there is much going on in your stomach and will want to purge some of that food in some way to help empty it; hence, the feeling of vomiting.

Drink plenty of fluids because you are losing much of it every time you vomit. You can also eat some fruits such as apples and bananas to prevent vomiting. If the vomiting becomes frequent, visit your doctor for possible IV hydration and medication.

Your Baby's Development

Your baby is growing very fast and looks like a tailed tadpole. Your baby's skeleton has begun to take shape and vital organs such as the circulatory system, muscles, bones, and the heart are developing quickly. The heart will start to separate into four chambers and some ultrasounds will notice your baby's heartbeat.

The brain and the spinal cord, which develop from the neural tube, have started to form. Other body parts like the fingers, nose, mouth, eyes, ears, and toes have started to show. The placenta and the umbilical cord, through which your baby receives nourishment continues to develop.

Week 6

Your baby is one month old and the growth and development process is still ongoing.

Changes In Your Body

At this stage, because of the positive pregnancy test results and the many symptoms bound to manifest this week, you are 100 percent sure of your pregnancy. Some of these signs and symptoms include:

Headache: If you do not drink enough fluids, or if you are anemic, you may experience headaches during your 6th week of pregnancy. In addition, the increased levels of progesterone can lead to headaches because migraines become less frequent as pregnancy progresses. Because of the fluctuating hormone production, your headache may worsen day-by-day.

If you experience this symptom, drink plenty of fluids, have a bottle of water with you every time, and if you are anemic, get your blood checked so you may get the right medication. If your headache persists or becomes severe, consult your doctor or OB.

Mood swings: This symptom is very common in most pregnant women. Pregnancy mood swings come from fatigue, physical stress, or the increased production of progesterone and estrogen

Understand that what you are experiencing is normal and will soon pass. To manage your stress level that can lead to mood swings, make sure that you get enough sleep, eat a balanced diet, and spend time with your partner and friends.

Smell sensitivity: You will notice that you want to smell any food before you take it or feel irritated by your friend's cologne. This symptom is one that many pregnant women experience. Researchers have speculated that it is a way of protecting your baby from harmful toxins because when you develop the habit of 'smelling your food'; you will not end up eating tainted or spoiled foods that can harm your baby.

Other than making sure you eat clean, well-cooked food, you can do very little about your heightened sense of smell: enjoy it.

Anxiety and Depression: It is normal to have a degree of worry about your pregnancy. You may start feeling anxious about your baby or yourself. For instance, you may start worrying about how you will look in 3 months or after birth, the weight, and height of your baby at birth and other worries out of your control.

It is OK to worry a little; however, if the worry becomes persistent and you find it hard to function normally, you need to see your OB immediately because anxiety and depression can lead to premature birth, low birth weight, miscarriage and suicide.

Because of the growing baby, you may gain or lose weight because of the continued vomiting and nausea. In the first trimester, it is normal to experience either weight gain or loss because people are different and their bodies react differently to the baby.

Your Baby's Development

Your baby is a quarter inch long and looks like a lentil.

The mouth, nose, ears eyes, legs, and arms have begun to take shape. In an ultrasound, you will notice a large head with black spots that mark your baby's eyes and nostrils, small depressions on the side of his/her head that mark your baby's ears, and protruding buds that mark your baby's legs and arms.

Your baby's heart beat is about 100 to 160 times per minute. The tissues that develop into the lungs appear and begin to form. During this week is when intestines and pituitary glands start to form. Other vital organs like muscles and bones are forming, and complex components of the brain are developing.

Your baby will start its movements but they will be very gentle that you will not be able to feel them.

Week 7

You are midway through your first trimester and your baby is really growing.

Changes In Your Body

At this stage, you are probably not showing because your baby is too small, but bloating can cause swelling in your lower abdomen. During this week, your mucous plug will develop from the cervical canal so that it can seal off the uterus for protection.

On the seventh week, depending on your vomiting and nausea persistence, you may start to gain weight. New symptoms you may notice during this week include:

Frequent urination: Your swelling uterus will place pressure on your bladder; because of the pressed bladder, you will feel the frequent need to use the restrooms. Also, the extra blood (from your baby) flowing to your kidneys will cause them to produce more urine.

If a burning sensation, or any sign of infection accompanies this symptom, immediately inform your doctor or OB.

Vaginal discharge: During this week, it is common to experience more vaginal discharge. You will notice more milky, odorless, or mild-smelling discharge on your pants. This happens because of the increased production of estrogen in your body and the increased blood flow to your vaginal area.

If your discharge is yellow, green, or gray in color, has unpleasant odor and causes you any discomfort such as itching, soreness, burning, and pain when urinating, visit your doctor immediately because this can be an infection.

Cravings and unusual hunger: Your body is working hard to ensure the baby grows and that is why you will feel hungrier than usual. You will also start to crave for foods you have never thought of eating or want to eat your favorite snack more often.

It's OK to feed your craving as long as what you eat is safe for you and your baby and make sure you do not eat too much of the unhealthy foods. If you crave foods rich in vitamins, avoid them or take very little because you are not supposed to overtake vitamins.

Your Baby's Development

Your baby has doubled in size since last week; at week 7, your baby is half an inch long. This week will see your child develop their blood type and the liver starts to produce red blood cells.

Appendix, pancreas, and intestines have fully formed and other organs such as the brain, bones, and the muscles are rapidly developing. Fingers and toes are emerging from the developing arms and legs are visible as paddles in ultrasound. The mouth, eyes, ears, and nose are also beginning to come into focus.

Week 8

At the 8th week, you will get your first ultrasound and will see your baby for the first time.

Changes In Your Body

Your breasts are still growing bigger week by week and you have to make sure you have the right-sized bra for support. In addition, a thick yellowish substance (colostrum) will discharge from your nipple.

You will feel bone-deep fatigue because your body is working extra hard to create a new human being. You can get a massage and exercise to help reduce this pain. Aversion to certain foods and smell sensitivity go on high alert because you will want to protect your baby from toxins. Your uterus is growing as your baby grows and because of this, you may experience cramping.

Your Baby's Development

Your baby is approximately an inch long, weighs close to 3 grams, and is at the end of the embryotic stage, is ready to become a fetus and due to this, the embryonic tail starts to disappear. Intestines protrude into the umbilical cord because they have grown longer and cannot fit in the abdomen. Bones start to harden and joints start taking shape.

Gonads start to form into either ovaries or testicles but you will not be able to know the sex of your baby just yet. Also, webbed fingers and toes begin to grow separate and longer and if you look closely, you can almost count them, eyelids have formed and cover the eyes, and breathing tubes extend from the throat to the branches of the developing lungs.

The mouth, jawline, and nose are clearly visible, ears are growing and sharing both internally and externally, and the teeth have formed.

Week 9

You and your baby are going through many rapid changes.

Changes In Your Body

You many notice that your waist has started thickening, but you still may not look pregnant. You may start to gain weight not because of the baby, but because of water retention.

The common pregnancy symptoms apparent during this week include mood swings, which are perfectly normal because of the increased production of hormones in your body. Other symptoms include bloating, morning sickness, fatigue, aches and pains.

You may find yourself sweating while others around you are shivering, this is also normal; it comes from the extra blood pumping throughout your body.

Your Baby's Development

Your baby is still an inch long and weighs about 3 grams just like the previous week, but for the first time, looks practically human because all the physical features such as legs, hands and head are clear. The baby's eyes have fully formed and the eyelids will remain closed until the 27th week.

Your baby is out of the embryotic stage and started the fetal stage. Because of this, the embryonic tail will completely disappear and the muscles and organs will start functioning on their own.

External sex organs are still developing but your doctor cannot distinguish them. The placenta has developed and can now take over the critical job of producing hormones.

Week 10

Your baby is now in the fetal stage and most of the critical weeks of development are over.

Changes In Your Body

At the tenth week, your pregnancy will still not show. Your uterus is becoming big as your baby grows and you will have gained some weight. You will still experience some bloating but other early pregnancy symptoms such as morning sickness and mood swings will subside.

Your Baby's Development

During your prenatal visits, you will be able to hear your baby's heartbeat and see his/her dramatic movement. Vital organs such as the kidney, liver, lungs, intestines, and brain have formed, started functioning, and will continue developing throughout your pregnancy.

Also toenails and fingernails have started to form and hair has begun to grow.

Week 11

At week 11, you and your baby are experiencing many changes.

Changes In Your Body

Slowly-by-slowly, you are gaining weight, but the good thing is that some of the early symptoms such as nausea, and vomiting are reducing and you are feeling more energetic now. Unfortunately, you are likely to experience symptoms like bloating, heartburn, and constipation because of the production of pregnancy hormones. You may notice changes in your fingernails, hair, and toenails. Again, is partly because of the increased hormone level in your body.

Your Baby's Development

Your baby is 1.5 inches long and about the size of a fig where the head makes up half of the size. Fingers and toes are separated and clear, bones are still hardening, and the skin is still transparent.

Your baby is learning how to swallow during this week and more blood vessels will appear in the placenta to provide the baby with oxygen and nutrients needed for growth. The ears will move from the neck to the side of the head.

Week 12

It is 3 months down the line. You can now be free and secure to tell friends and family members of the good news because chances of miscarriage have decreased.

Changes In Your Body

Your uterus, which is almost big enough to fill your pelvis, protrudes above your pubic bone and you will start showing. Your body is beginning to adjust to changes in hormonal level and many of the early pregnancy symptoms completely subside. Because of increased production of progesterone, you will experience heartburn and mood swings.

You may start having dark brown patches of skin on your face and spots around your body. This can be treated by taking some Vitamin A and as stated earlier, you are not supposed to take large doses of vitamin A because it can damage some parts of your baby; parts such as the liver.

Your Baby's Development

Your baby is 2.8 inches long and weighs about half an ounce. During this week, your baby will start to clench and open fists, bend his/her arms, clench eyes, make sucking movements with his/her mouth, and twist elbows and wrist.

Intestines will move into the abdominal cavity and kidneys will start excreting urine into the bladder. Nerve cells multiply rapidly and the brain, which is still developing, starts to produce its own hormones. Muscles begin to respond to the brain.

Week 13

At week 13, you are at the end of your first trimester where most of the critical development occurs.

Changes In Your Body

Your early pregnancy symptoms are easing and you feel more energetic. Your uterus grows up and out of your pelvic bone announcing to the world that you are pregnant and most importantly, relieves pressure from your bladder. You can start wearing slightly larger clothes since your favorite pair of jeans or skirt may become uncomfortable.

Your waistline thickens and you may begin to experience severe abdominal pains or ligament pain that occurs when ligaments stretch and pull. You may also experience heartburns. Because of the production of colostrum, your breasts are still developing and becoming more sensitive.

Your Baby's Development

Your baby is almost 3 inches long and weighs about an ounce. Veins are clearly visible through the still thin skin, and the baby is learning how to catch up with the head that is a third of the body.

All physical features are formed and in the right place.

Diet And Fitness For The First Trimester

As you have seen, the first trimester is critically important. This means you should eat and exercise right. Here are the things you should get right:

If you have not been taking **prenatal vitamin**, start taking them. The vitamins you should be taking include vitamins rich in Folic acid, Calcium, and Iron. Folic acid aids in the prevention of neural tube defects, which are very serious conditions that can cause brain and spinal cord abnormalities in your baby. Calcium helps your baby develop healthy and strong bones and teeth, while Iron helps your baby's growth and development by providing oxygen to the baby and preventing you from developing anemia.

You can buy these prenatal vitamins as over-the-counter medication where the pharmacist will prescribe the amount to take. In addition, these vitamins are present in foods and fluids such as milk, green vegetables and liver.

Other prenatal vitamins you should start taking are vitamin A, vitamin C and vitamin E. Vitamin A helps your baby's embryonic growth such as circulatory system, respiratory system, lungs, kidneys, and eyes development. Taking large amounts of vitamin A can be harmful to your baby because the development only needs a few grams.

Some of the ways taking large amounts of vitamin A can negatively affect the baby include malformation of the skull, lungs, heart, and the eyes. To prevent this, take about 0.6mg of vitamin A in a day and don't eat liver and any liver products more than once in a week because they are very rich in vitamin A.

Vitamin C: You and your baby need vitamin C daily because it helps the body create collagen, a structural protein in the baby's body that is an important component of tendons, bones, skin, and cartilage. Lack of vitamin C can cause mental impairment in your unborn baby.

Pregnant women of different ages will require different amounts of vitamin C. If you are 18 years and below, take 80mg of vitamin C per day, and if you are 19 years and above, take 85mg daily.

Copper: This is a mineral found in both plants and animals. It helps in red blood cells formation in your body especially now when your blood supply has doubled. It will also help in formation of your baby's heart, blood vessels, nervous system, and skeletal system. You only need 1 mg (milligram) of copper per day.

Vitamin E: Vitamin E is a fatty soluble substance mostly found in olive oil. The main function of vitamin E is to help protect your baby's multiplying cells membranes, maintain their structure. Vitamin E plays a key role in the development of your baby's lungs. It helps maintain healthy blood sugar levels.

Eat a variety of foods daily to get all the nutrients you and your baby need. Ensure that every meal you eat contains starch, proteins, vegetables, and average amount of vitamins (indicated above). All these nutrients will ensure that you stay healthy and that your baby grows healthy and strong. Ask your doctor or OB about the foods you should and should not take for the safety of your baby and let him/her review the set amount of vitamins you take in a day to ensure that you take the correct amount.

Have a daily exercise routine throughout your pregnancy. This is because exercise will help you maintain a healthy weight, maintain an upright posture, build stamina needed during labor and delivery, and decrease some pregnancy symptoms such as fatigue and backaches. Find qualified and registered persons who have experience teaching pregnant woman Pilates and yoga poses for strengthening and toning. Jogging, swimming, brisk walking, and cycling, are some of the good and safe forms of exercise you can vary and do every day for a period of 20 to 30 minutes. Before you start a new exercise routine, let your doctor know.

Avoid all drugs whether legal or illegal, skin creams such as acne medication and beverages that contain caffeine. If you want to use any medication or drug, visit your doctor to get medication that will not affect your baby. If you have any kind of medical appointment, inform your doctor that you are expectant. He/she has to be aware because some medications are not ideal prescriptions for pregnant women.

Drink plenty of fluids every day to prevent dehydration and avoid some pregnancy symptoms like fainting and dizziness.

Stop bad habits such as smoking and drinking. Consult your doctor for guidance if you find it hard to quit because these substances can cause defects and abnormalities to your growing baby.

Learn side sleeping by hugging a pillow and wrapping your legs around it or putting pillows around you to prevent you from rolling on your back. This will help you choose a comfortable sleeping position as your belly grows.

What To Expect In The Second Trimester

The second trimester is the period from week 14 all through to week 27 of pregnancy. You will notice that you don't experience many of the early symptoms of pregnancy like nausea, vomiting, and fatigue. The common name for the second trimester is "the honeymoon stage" because you will not experience many symptoms common in the previous trimester.

Week 14

In the 14th week of pregnancy, and the first week of your second trimester, you will feel relaxed because your body has adjusted to the internal changes taking place.

Changes In Your Body

Although most of the symptoms have disappeared, your mood swings will tend to increase week by week during this trimester and breasts will continue to grow. Your waistline will also continue to expand, and you will still continue gaining weight.

Spots on your body will continue to darken and new moles may develop.

Your Baby's Development

Your baby is between two and three inches long, weighs about 1.5 ounces, is still moving, but you cannot feel the kicks and movements yet. Major developments during this week are your baby's liver will start to produce bile, and the spleen will start to produce red blood cells. Eyes continue to draw closer to one another and as the neck grows longer, the chin lifts from the chest.

During this week, your baby will start to suck his/her thumb and make facial expressions such as frowning, grimacing, and squinting. Moreover, the kidney will start to produce urine that will pass through the amniotic fluid, and your baby will start to draw its nutrients directly from the placenta.

Week 15

Your baby is still growing and now that many of the symptoms have disappeared, you can now enjoy being pregnant.

Changes In Your Body

During this week, you will not experience many changes and symptoms. Your baby is growing and this causes your uterus to grow; due to this, you will experience sharp pains in the abdomen because the ligaments that support your uterus are stretching.

By the 15th week, you have gained around 6 pounds or less.

Your Baby's Development

Your baby is still growing and by now, he/she is 4 inches long and about 1.75 pounds with the head being the biggest part.

A fine hair called lanugo will develop and cover your baby's skin to help the baby maintain a constant temperature. This hair will be present throughout your pregnancy and will disappear during birth.

Bones are still hardening and the brain is still developing. Your baby's muscle reflexes cause movements, but you are yet to feel or hear them. Parts like legs, hands, neck, toenails, and fingernails are growing longer every day. In addition, your baby will start hearing sounds like your heartbeat and breathing.

Week 16

At week 16, your baby is about 4-5 inches, and weighs approximately four ounces. Your baby's muscles and backbone are becoming stronger, and your baby can substantially straighten his or her neck and head.

At this stage, your baby's eyes are working, can perceive light, and make small side-to-side movements; however, your baby's eyelids are still tightly shut.

At week 16, some of the changes you should expect include:

Changes In Your Body

Milk glands will start their function, which is to produce milk for the baby as early as now, and because of the increased blood flow, the veins around your breasts will become more visible. Your breasts are still tender, swollen, and more sensitive.

Constipation and heartburn may still be present, and you may start to nosebleed. Nosebleeds occur when the tiny blood vessels in your nose rupture due to the increased blood flow; this is usually harmless. However, if it persists, consult your doctor.

Due to the increasingly active hormones in your body, your skin may look oiler and shiner, and the increase in blood flow to your body may make your face look brighter. At week 16, you will still experience cravings.

Your Baby's Development

As stated, during the 16th week, your baby is about 4-4.75-5 inches long and weighs about 3.9-4 ounces. Parts like the eyes and the ears have settled into their permanent position and the facial muscles are continuing to develop.

Your baby's genitals are fully developed and your doctor can distinguish if your baby is a boy or a girl. Your baby's visual sensitivity development will show some progress because your baby will use his or her hands to protect his/her eyes. Fat that acts like insulation will begin to build underneath the skin and the circulatory and urinary systems are now functioning.

Week 17

Some of the things you should expect include:

Changes In Your Body

Now you look more like a pregnant woman because your uterus has protruded and you can feel it. When you stand, your uterus moves to the sides and your abdomen has grown to provide space for your growing baby.

Pain in the legs (sciatic nerve pain) and back may start to occur and to alleviate them, avoid standing in one place for a long time and use pillows for support when seated. You will also experience heartburns, mood swings, and constipation.

You are still gaining weight week-by-week, and you should have gained around 5 to 20 pounds depending on your initial weight.

Your Baby's Development

Your baby is still growing; he or she is about 5.5 inches and 5 ounces; the skeleton, previously made up of soft cartilage is now developing into solid bones. Umbilical cord and placenta are still growing in length, thickness, and strength.

Bones have fully formed but will remain flexible to allow for passage through the birth canal and the head is no longer big and your baby has started looking like a normal baby.

Week 18

At week 18, you are still in the honeymoon phase. Here are the changes you should expect:

Changes In Your Body

As your belly stretches and your waistline expands, stretch marks will become more prominent. You are still gaining weight and again, this will differ from one mom to another.

Symptoms such as constipation, heartburn, frequent urination, and pains in the leg and back are still present. Other symptoms you may experience during this week include:

Feeling dizzy and faint: The increased production of the hormone progesterone can lead to lightheadedness and make blood vessels dilate, causing lower blood pressure. The blood diverted to the uterus will take longer than normal to make its way back to your brain and you are likely to faint when you stand up. You can solve this symptom by drinking plenty of fluids to maintain steady blood pressure and eat a balanced diet every 3 to 4 hours to keep a stable blood sugar level.

Do not abruptly leap out of bed or off the couch; move slowly and when you feel faint, sit down with your head between your knees. Itchiness in the abdomen, hands, or feet is common and resolves after birth. A moisturizing cream may help reduce this feeling.

Your Baby's Development

Your baby is 5.5 inches long and about 7 ounces. Bones and inner ears are still hardening and hearing has become better. The brain part that receives and sends nerve signals is still developing and your baby will start reacting to loud noise.

If you are having a girl, the fallopian tube and uterus will start to develop and move to the correct position.

Week 19

Here is what to expect at week 19:

Changes In Your Body

You may start having dry skin because of increased blood flow and metabolism. Use gentle lotions, eat well-balanced meals, and drink plenty of fluids to prevent this problem.

If your weight gain is on track, by the end of this week, you should have gained an average of 7 to 16 pounds. Your breasts are still growing, and you may start noticing a dark line running down the middle of your stomach (linea nigra) which fades away some months after delivery.

Your Baby's Development

Although your baby is becoming more active as bones continue to develop, your baby will be asleep for around 20 hours a day. He/she is about 7 inches and 7 ounces.

The arms and legs are now proportional to the body and sensory parts of the brain are still developing.

Week 20

At week 20, you are at the middle of your pregnancy having survived all the early symptoms of pregnancy.

Changes In Your Body

You will still experience symptoms such as fatigue, pains, constipation, itching, frequent urination, and heartburn, but the good news is that you will start feeling your baby's jabs and pokes as he/she moves around your uterus.

Your belly and waistline are still growing and you may start getting stares from strangers; brush them off and be proud because you are really doing a great job.

Your Baby's Development

By now, your baby is about 7 inches long and weighs about 11 ounces. Lanugo has started covering your entire baby and vernix, which shields your baby from the amniotic fluid, has started forming. Hair on the scalp is still growing and the lungs are still forming but your baby can breathe. Ears are formed and functioning on their own.

Week 21

You are now in week 21 and many changes are still happening

Changes In Your Body

You are becoming bigger as your baby grows. Your pregnancy is very noticeable and you should have started wearing maternity clothes or large clothes to accommodate your belly. Your legs and thighs may start to swell and pains/aches are still present. Use pregnancy or regular pillow to elevate your legs and reduce swelling.

Other symptoms you will suffer from are constipation, fatigue, frequent urination, heartburn, and increased appetite.

Your Baby's Development

Your baby is about the size of a banana, weighs about 11 ounces, and is almost 8 inches long. The umbilical cord is still strengthening and getting longer; the digestive system is also developing and has started practicing its function using the amniotic fluid, which your baby swallows regularly.

Body parts such as the eyelids, toenails, fingernails and eyebrows are fully developed and the circulatory system is also functioning.

Week 22

Here is what to expect once you hit week 22:

Changes In Your Body

Your uterus is growing; it is now about 2 centimeters above your belly button. By now, you should have gained about 10 to 20 pounds. Most of the pregnancy discomforts have disappeared but unfortunately, you will continue to suffer from some of them such as vaginal discharge, constipation, and pains all throughout your pregnancy.

You may start experiencing Braxton-hick contractions, which are usually mild and unpredictable. It is normal because this is early preparation for labor; if the pains persist, inform your doctor.

Your Baby's Development

Your baby is growing fast and is the size of a papaya, weighing about a pound and almost 11 inches long. The eyes have fully formed but the irises do not have any pigment yet. The Sensory system is also developing and your baby has started exercising his/her sense of touch and if you look at him or her in an ultrasound, you will notice your baby rubbing his face, legs, and neck.

The liver has started producing enzymes required for the breakdown of bilirubin, but your liver will have to assist your baby's liver by getting rid of the bilirubin because your baby's red blood cells have a short life span. If you are having a girl, the ovaries, egg cells, uterus, and fallopian tube have fully formed.

Week 23

At week 23, below should be your expectations:

Changes In Your Body

Other than the growing uterus, weight gain and breast enlargement, there are no major changes in your body. Symptoms like swollen legs and thighs, vaginal discharge, frequent urination are still present.

Your Baby's Development

Your baby's lungs are still developing; however, they are not yet ready to work on their own. The Lanugo, which may become darker, has covered your baby's body and the skin remains loose. Fat and pigmentation starts to form during this week.

Your baby is also moving, and you may feel punches and kicks. Your baby now resembles a little doll, weighs a little more than a pound, and is nearing one foot in length.

Week 24

Week 24 brings many changes such as:

Changes In Your Body

Although you have 16 weeks to go, your breasts may start producing colostrum as early as now, a situation that will continue. Remember people are different and if you do not notice the colostrum, it is still OK.

Braxton-hick contractions are still present, but if their frequency and pain has increased, contact your doctor. By this week, you should have gained between 12 to 24 pounds but again, moms are different. Let your doctor determine if your weight gain is healthy.

Because of the swelling of the mucous membranes, you may experience nasal congestion and cold symptoms. You may experience blurred vision and dry eyes, but these are usually not common and cannot cause any major hindrance.

Your Baby's Development

The baby's brain is still developing and the lungs have begun to develop branches and cells that produce surfactant. Your baby's eyes are still shut. Hair on the scalp, taste buds, eyelashes, eyebrows, and arms are still developing at an even pace.

Your baby weighs about 1.2 pounds and is almost a foot tall.

Note: Undergo a glucose test to screen for gestation diabetes that tends to occur during this time; this should not worry you because it disappears after birth. Gestation diabetes births from a lack of enough insulin in your body to metabolize sugar in the bloodstream.

Week 25

Here is what to expect once you hit week 25:

Changes In Your Body

As your baby grows, you are also becoming bigger. Your belly is protruding and your breasts are still growing. You may notice that your hair is growing but chances are it will fall off after birth. You are likely to suffer from constipation, weight gain, backaches, and pain in the legs, itchiness, and heartburn.

Your Baby's Development

Your baby is over 1.5 pounds and about 13.5 inches tall. Your baby is making many movements during this stage but do not worry because that is a good thing.

The good news is, during this week, your baby will start to plump up as fat builds under the skin which is still developing. In ultrasounds, your baby will look more like a person compared to the previous weeks.

Week 26

You made through the second trimester; you are days away from entering your third trimester: the last stage of your pregnancy.

Changes In Your Body

At week 26, you will feel more back pain because of the increased weight (14 to 28 pounds) but try not to weigh yourself daily or more than once in a day because your weight will fluctuate due to water retention.

Braxton-hicks contractions will become more frequent and will feel like menstrual cramps. You may begin to experience pain under your ribs caused by your baby's kicks and stretches. You will still experience frequent urination and constipation.

Your Baby's Development

Many things will happen during this week; your baby will be around 14 inches tall and 2 pounds. This week will see your baby open his/her eyes and blink for the first time. The lungs are still developing, and your baby continues to breathe in and out the amniotic fluid as blood vessels develop around them.

The nervous system is also developing and your baby can differentiate your voice from others around you. Fat is building up underneath the baby's skin and will do so until you deliver. The umbilical cord is still growing thicker and stronger as it provides your baby with the necessary nutrients.

If you are having a boy, this week sees the baby's testicles move into the scrotum.

Diet And Fitness For The Second Trimester

All through pregnancy, the idea should be to eat a balanced diet. However, here are diet and fitness tips for your second trimester:

*Be very careful about what you eat during this trimester because anything you eat also goes to the baby. Your appetite will increase and you will feel as if you have to eat for two; instead of eating large one-of-meals, eat small frequent portions of well-balanced meals. A balanced diet will provide your baby with the nutrients he or she needs to grow healthy and develop. Further, a balanced diet will keep you healthy.

*If at any point, you feel like you have gained too much weight, just continue exercising, and do not try any sort of diet because this may deny your baby some of the important growth and development nutrients.

*Continue drinking plenty of fluids to prevent dehydration that can lead to fatigue, shortness of breath, and dizziness. You should avoid artificial fluids such as sodas and sweet beverages because they will cause dehydration. Stay away from caffeine as much as possible because it raises blood pressure. Water, vegetable/fruit juices, and milk are the best fluids to take during your pregnancy.

***Exercise** for at least 30 minutes every day and get a massage to help you relax and relieve some pains and aches.

*If your pregnancy is healthy and your doctors have not advised you otherwise, sex is still safe for you and your baby. You might find yourself enjoying it more than ever before because of the increased blood flow.

*You can use cocoa butter to prevent or reduce stretch marks that may occur during this trimester because of the expanding waistline and growing belly.

*Forget about high heels until you give birth: stick to flats because your protruding belly will change your center of gravity and you are likely to lose balance when you wear high heels

*If you are craving salty foods, eat string cheese, and if you are craving sweet foods, reach for **yoghurt or fruits** instead of sweets and candy bars. This way you, will stick to a healthy diet and deal with your cravings.

What To Expect In The Third Trimester

The third trimester is the period from the 27th week of pregnancy to delivery.

Week 27

In the first week of your third trimester, here is what to expect:

Changes In Your Body

By now, you should have gained a total of 15 to 30 pounds. The common symptoms during this stage are constipation, heartburn, fatigue, Braxton-hicks contraction, frequent urination, pains, and aches in the legs, abdomen, and back.

Note: Depending on your blood type, your doctor may administer an Rh immune globulin shot to prevent antibodies from harming your baby.

Your Baby's Development

You might have noticed that for the last trimester (2nd trimester), your baby's growth was slow, but as the third trimester begins, your baby will grow at a faster rate. At week 27, your baby is about 15 inches long and weighs over 2 pounds.

Layers of retina start forming. Lungs are still developing and as your baby learns to inhale and exhale using the amniotic fluid, he/she may experience hiccups.

Week 28

Here is what to expect in week 28:

Changes In Your Body

You may have a hard time eating large meals, or may at times 'not feel hungry'. This happens because your baby and uterus are taking up quite some room. Eating small meals frequently will be of great help. Weight gain by the end of this week should be 16 to 32 pounds.

Symptoms like pains in the abdomen, constipation, heartburn, and Braxton-hicks contraction become more frequent.

Your Baby's Development

At week 28, your baby weighs close to 4 pounds and about 6 inches in length. The deep ridges and indentations in the brain also start to develop. Eyelids are partly open and eyelashes become visible. Movements, kicks, and punches become more frequent.

If you were to deliver now (though premature), your baby has 90 percent chances of survival without any physical disability or impairment.

Week 29

At week 29, you are nearing the last 10 weeks of your pregnancy. Here is what to brace for:

Changes In Your Body

You will still experience last weeks' symptoms such as itchiness, mood swings, and food cravings; this is normal. Pains in the ribs and difficulty breathing will become severe because your baby's kicks and punches become hard and frequent.

Varicose veins may start to form on your legs but you can use compression stockings to elevate your feet, thus minimizing this symptom.

Your Baby's Development

Your baby is the size of a butternut squash and organs like the brain, lungs, and muscles are still developing. If you are having a boy, the testes will probably start to descend from the abdomen to the scrotum.

Your baby is making more and more blood for use and this means you should increase your level of iron intake to around 30 milligrams per day unless directed otherwise.

Week 30

You may feel that your pregnancy is endless, but do not worry, you only have about 10 weeks to go.

Changes In Your Body

Your weight is increasing week-by-week, your beautiful belly is very big, and your waistline has increased. You may feel extra tired, but having learnt new sitting, standing, walking, and sleeping positions, you will survive this feeling.

You should have gained between 18 and 35 pounds by the end of this week. During these last weeks, weight gain slows down for some women, this is normal; however, if you completely stop gaining weight, talk to your doctor.

Your Baby's Development

Although your baby spends most of the time sleeping, he/she is getting used to his/her sleeping and waking routine and is becoming very active while awake.

Wrinkles in your baby's skin will start to smooth out as the fat underneath it continues to build. By now, the digestive system has formed and is fully functional. The lungs and brain are still developing and learning how to function on their own. Your baby's hearing has greatly improved.

Week 31

As you start your 31st week, here is what to expect:

Changes In Your Body

At week 31, you may find it impossible to find a comfortable sleeping position especially if you are sleeping for long periods; use pillows or special pregnancy pillows to find a comfortable sleeping. You should not sleep on your belly or back.

Your ligament pain may decrease during this week, but back pains will become severe. From this week onwards, you may start leaking urine when you laugh, cough, or sneeze; this is perfectly normal. Doing Kegel exercises may help prevent or minimize this.

Colostrum is still leaking; you can buy nipple shields to avoid messing your clothes. For some moms, this discharge may never leak during pregnancy, which is normal and the colostrum will appear after birth.

Your Baby's Development

Your baby is growing longer and heavier day-by-day and by this week, your baby is over half the size and weight he/she will be at birth.

By week 31, body parts such as the eyes, ears, toenails, fingernails, mouth, fingers, and toes have completed developing and can function. The breathing system, nervous system, and digestive system are almost mature.

Week 32

8 more weeks to go! At week 32, brace for:

Changes In Your Body

During this week, your body will see no major changes other than increased weight gain and a growing belly. You will also experience symptoms present in the previous week and they will become more frequent and severe as you near your due date.

Your Baby's Development

Your baby is around 17 inches long and weighs about 4.5 pounds. The brain is still developing, the bones have fully formed; however, they are still soft and flexible. The skeleton has fully formed.

During this week or later in your pregnancy, your baby will start to dream and due to this, he/she will start sleeping in segments of 20-40 minutes. This will disrupt your sleep. Beginning this week, your baby will seem less active because he/she has grown and there is less room in your womb for movements.

Moreover, your baby may turn to a head-down position, but if your baby has not turned by the end of the week, do not worry, he/she well turn sometime before birth. If he/she does not turn, you may have to deliver through a C-section.

Week 33

The countdown has started and you have just 7 weeks to go. Week 33 will bring along these changes:

Changes In Your Body

By the end of this week, you should have gained between 21 and 35 pounds if your pregnancy is healthy. Your belly is the size of a basketball. One of the common symptoms you will experience more frequently during this week is insomnia. This is because you and your baby have different sleeping schedules.

Your heart may skip beats at times, which is normal because it has to pump faster to accommodate the increased blood, which has increased by more than 40 percent. If this symptom happens frequently, inform your doctor.

Your Baby's Development

At about 17 inches long, your baby is still growing and gaining weight as fat builds underneath the skin. From this week onwards, you will notice that your baby is not moving much and will spend most of the time sleeping because there is less room now. The kicks and punches will become a bit more painful because your baby is growing and can really kick harder.

All bones continue to harden except the skull. The lungs are still practicing to accommodate your baby's breathing patterns after birth. If your baby is not in the head-down position, do not worry, you have seven more weeks to go.

Week 34

At week 34, you may feel as if you have been pregnant for years; relax, you have less than two months to go.

Changes In Your Body

As your baby grows, your uterus is still growing and the level of amniotic fluid produced increases. Excess amniotic fluid absorbs into your body. Your uterus is about 5.5 inches above your belly button. The belly button may become sensitive, place a bandage over it to avoid irritation. By week 34, you should have gained around 22- 35 pounds. You may notice a reduction of pressure on your lungs and chest during this week because your baby will move down to the pelvic area.

Due to the relaxation of muscles in the lower esophagus, heartburns will become more persistent. Because of the increased retention of water in your body, your hands, feet, wrists, and face may swell. If headache, dizziness and abdominal pains, accompany the swelling, contact your doctor. In order to reduce this symptom, drink plenty of water and soak your hands and legs in warm water.

Your Baby's Development

At about 17.5 inches and weighing close to 5 pounds, most of your baby's organs are almost at full maturity (except the lungs). Your baby's legs are bent and held near the trunk because by now, there is less room in your womb.

Your baby's pupils are developed and can dilate and constrict in response to light. With the help of the fat stored under the skin, your baby can now regulate his/ her temperature. In addition, the lanugo that covered your baby will start disappearing.

Week 35

Five more weeks to go; here is what week 35 of pregnancy has in store for you:

Changes In Your Body

Your uterus is about 6 inches above your belly button. You may be able to see your belly button shift, which is normal. You may experience back pain, pelvic pain, and pelvic numbness. This numbness comes from the pressure on the pelvic nerves and can continue until birth. Because of the increased pressure on your bladder, you will urinate more often.

By now, you have probably gained 25 to 30 pounds, and you may or may not gain more weight in the remaining weeks. You may feel stressed and anxious about your baby's arrival, which is normal to most pregnant mom. To ease your mind, try talking to someone who has been in this position before.

Your Baby's Development

At approximately 18 inches and 6 pounds, your baby will continue to put on weight. Most of the organs like the liver and kidney are fully formed and functioning on their own.

The lanugo will continue to disappear and a fine vellus hair will start to grow to replace it. If you deliver in this week, your baby will need specialized care because he/she will still be premature. Chances of survival are very good but the baby will be at risk of having breathing problems and jaundice.

Week 36

During this week, you should undergo Group B streptococcus screening. This screening will help determine if you have this type of bacteria so your medic can treat you with antibiotics during labor to prevent infecting your baby because it can cause serious lung infections.

Changes In Your Body

During this week, you may experience high blood sugar levels and high blood pressure. You may also suffer from UTIs because of hemorrhoids and frequent urination. You can ask your doctor to prescribe a cream to help with the hemorrhoids, but you still cannot do much about the urination.

You may feel your baby rest on your pelvic bone, this is normal. Symptoms such as insomnia, constipation, fatigue, Braxton-hicks contractions, back pains, and restlessness are still present and may continue until your delivery day.

Your Baby's Development

During this week, your baby is "last preterm" and is about 18 inches in length, weighing about 6 pounds. Your baby has pretty much finished growing.

Week 37

Here you are, at the ninth and final month of your pregnancy. Your doctor may want to meet you more than often during this week so he or she can track your progress and do the necessary and important screening.

Changes In Your Body

At this point, you have experienced very many symptoms and learnt to cope with them in one way or another. Because your baby is relatively big now, some symptoms such as swelling, aches, Braxton-hicks contraction, and pains may be very severe at this point; you will continue to experience them for the remaining week.

Your breasts have expanded, become sensitive, and are full of milk. Exhaustion is very common during this "full term" stage.

Your Baby's Development

Although the brain and lungs still need some more time to mature, most of the organs are fully developed and if born today, chances of surviving without any complication are good.

Your baby's hair is still growing depending on genetics. At week 37, the skin has become smoother and the Amniotic fluid has started to decrease because of the growing baby occupying a lot of the available space.

During this week, growth is very slow and by the end of it, your baby will weigh about 6.5 pounds.

Week 38

You made it to week 38. Here is what to expect:

Changes In Your Body

At week 38, you will have increased mucus discharge as your cervix softens preparing for birth. The last weeks of pregnancy do not see much weight gain, but symptoms present in the last week will persist.

Your Baby's Development

The only new and major development during this week is that tear ducts start to form. All organs have fully formed and are functioning, but since your baby is not yet born, he/she is still growing. Your baby should have turned into a head-down position (a process called engagement or lightening) and if not, let your doctor screen for breech and advice you on what to do.

Week 39

You are one week away from carrying your baby to full term. In week 39, brace for:

Changes In Your Body

In preparation for delivery, the cervix is becoming shorter, thinner, and softer. During this week, you are likely to experience discomforts and difficulty getting up from a sitting position.

You will still experience false labor contraction. You can differentiate false labor contraction from real labor contraction because false labor contraction will occur for seconds and disappear, but real labor contraction will occur for long period and will prevent you from walking or talking.

Your baby is moving closer to your cervix; if your water breaks during this week, call your doctor.

Your Baby's Development

Your baby is ready to come out. The lungs are fully mature but will not be able to function on their own until after birth. Although your baby is approximately 7 pounds, he or she is still growing. Your baby should remain active until birth and if not, contact your doctor.

Week 40

You made it to your last week of pregnancy and your baby will be out anytime from now, Congratulations mom. Although you might have one week or two to go, be prepared.

Changes In Your Body

This is a very exciting and challenging time for you as you anxiously await the arrival of your baby. During this week, pain will increase and you will feel more tired than before, which will make you want to stop engaging in all activities. Remember exercise or walk for 30 minutes every day.

Brixton-hicks contractions that prepare the cervix for delivery will become frequent but be careful not to confuse them will the real contraction. If the contractions become severe and occur for prolonged periods, may be it is your due date. Call your doctor.

A white substance will begin to secrete from your nipples and this is normal. It indicates that your body is prepared to feed your child after birth.

Your Baby's Development

Your baby is grown, mature, and ready to come to his/her new world. All organs are fully formed except the brain and the lungs which will continue to grow even after birth.

By this week your baby has moved near your cervix.

Diet And Exercise For The Third Trimester

Throughout this trimester, your baby is growing rapidly and will need more nutrients, As much as you feel like eating for two, maintain healthy eating habits at every meal, and drink plenty of fluids (especially water).

You may feel tired, but do not skip your 30 minutes exercise. This is the only way you can relax and strengthen your pelvic that has much pressure on it. Prenatal yoga classes can be very helpful but again, do not introduce a new exercise routine without consulting your doctor.

Get enough sleep. Because of the big belly, you may find it hard to sleep at night but sleep on your sides with your legs bent. Use a pillow to support your back and your belly.

Prenatal massages can reduce leg cramps and back pains.

Start your birth plan as early as the beginning of this trimester and include details about your preferences for the birth. Let your doctor tell you what to do in case of an emergency. You can also start childbirth classes; these classes will prepare you for labor and delivery and inform you about what to do to relief pain.

Bonus: How To Prepare For Labor And Delivery

Although it is hard to predict your due date, adequate preparation will help your birthing experience go as smoothly as possible. Some of the things you will need to do are:

Exercise

One of the best and mostly used exercises during pregnancy are Kegel exercises. With the help of your trainer, do Kegel exercises daily so you can strengthen your ligaments and pelvic muscles. Yoga exercises are also good because they will help release tension in your muscles. Always remember to consult your doctor before you try any new exercise.

Learn and Understand the Stages of Labor

You will go through three stages of labor; the duration taken in each stage will vary.

During the ***first labor***, muscles of the uterus will start to contract and relax. This will help to open the cervix to allow for the passage of your baby. The labor will start as irregular contractions that will last for less than a minute.

Later, you will experience active contractions that will be regular and will last for more than a minute. When the contractions become active, go to the hospital, or contact your doctor.

In your ***second stage***, the cervix is completely open and your baby will travel down and out of the birth canal.

The ***third stage*** of labor will occur after birth. You will experience contractions until the placenta comes out of your body.

Eating

During labor, you should consume plenty of fluids and light meals, or snacks such as a piece of toast, or popsicles. This will help keep your strength up as you go through the labor. Some recommended fluids include sports drink, fruit juice, chicken broth; however, let your doctor advice you on the best fluid for you.

Have a Birth Plan

A written or typed down birth plan will help you and your partner (if any) outline what you would like to happen during your labor and delivery. In the birth plan, include things like the name of your baby, your birthing environment, and pain management options. Let your doctor and partner have their copies.

Pain Management Options

Labor is painful and intense, but with your doctor's help, you can decide on which pain management option to go for and what level of pain you are going to bear before you get pain management options. Some of these pain management options are epidural, saddle block, Demerol, pudendal block, Nubain.

Decide Your Birthing Environment

You can choose to give birth at home, birthing center, or in the hospital. Let your doctor and partner help you decide the best place to deliver your baby. Although it provides you with a comfortable atmosphere for labor and delivery, a home birth can be risky. If you go with a home birth, seek the help of a midwife or someone who has experience with home birth.

If you decide to deliver at a hospital, look for a hospital near your home and visit the place some days earlier to familiarize yourself with the environment. In addition, choose the doctor you feel most comfortable with to help you during your delivery process.

Pack your hospital bag early

To avoid last minute rush and forgetting some of the important things, pack your hospital bag as early as possible (some days or even weeks before). Some of the things you will need in that bag are diapers, wet wipes, soft swaddles, soft baby clothes, and extra clean clothes for you.

Conclusion

Thank you again for downloading this book!

I hope this book was able to help you to know what to expect at every step of your pregnancy. With this information you can develop strategies to help you deal with some of the challenging pregnancy symptoms and enjoy your pregnancy.

Thank you and good luck!

Preview Of - Pregnancy: Expecting A Baby For New Moms

When that home pregnancy test kit or blood test returns positive, your world spines off. Immediately, you start thinking of all the things you out to buy, all the ways you ought to prepare, and all the changes you will undergo.

Amidst the excitement, it is normal to feel panicky because the thought of carrying a baby to term, taking care of your health as well as the health of the baby and caring for a baby after birth is overwhelming.

The best way to prepare yourself for motherhood as well as pregnancy is to become knowledgeable. In this guide, **Expecting a Baby for New Moms**, we shall look at, and understand the trimesters and the changes you can expect to see as your pregnancy progresses. You will also learn about how to take care of your health and your baby's as well as how to prepare for labor and child birth.

Enjoying Reading My Books? Maybe You Want To Read These Books Too

Below you'll find some of my other books that are on Amazon and Kindle as well. Simply click on the links below to check them out.

Want to know when next book is released? Subscribe here www.lacobiz.com

Pregnancy: Your Baby Guide Week For Week (not yet published)

Recommended:

Ketogenic Diet: Top 50 Breakfast Recipes

Ketogenic Diet: Top 50 Lunch Recipes

Yoga: Beginners Guide - For Yoga Poses - Easy Steps And Pictures

Mindfulness - Meditation For Beginners – Stress Free Body Depression And Anxiety Relief

5 Weeks Ketogenic Plan, Weight Loss Recipes - Easy Steps For beginners

Ketogenic: Ketogenic Diet - Mistakes Protection Handbook Smoothies Cleanse - Detox Diet And Lose Weight In A Healthy Way

Don't forget to subscribe to my newsletter! www.lacobiz.com

Made in the USA
San Bernardino, CA
02 December 2016